I0440406

The Day
Healthy Eating
Became an
Eating Disorder
Welcome to Life With
Orthorexia
Nervosa

The Day
Healthy Eating
became an
Eating Disorder
Welcome to Life With
ORTHOREXIA
NERVOSA

By M Fernandez

This book is dedicated to
healthy eaters everywhere.

Contents:

1.   What is orthorexia nervosa?
2.   How are people diagnosed?
3.   Who suffers from orthorexia
        nervosa?
4.   Where are the "correct appetite"
        people?
5.   What makes them different?
6.   Why do they eat this way?
7.   When did healthy eating
        become a disorder?
8.   What do healthy eaters have to
        fear?
9.   Is there hope?
10.   Who cares?

1. What is Orthorexia Nervosa?

According to recently published news reports, the American Psychiatric Association (APA) is attempting to have orthorexia ("correct diet") nervosa (ON) recognized as an eating disorder or mental disorder.

The term orthorexia nervosa was first coined by British doctor, Steven Bratman, in 1997. In early 2015, the APA began to push for an official diagnosis.

There is no known biological cause for orthorexia nervosa.

Headlines stating that, "Healthy Eating Said to be a Mental Disorder" are incorrect. That is not an accurate assessment of the actual disorder. It isn't a healthy eating lifestyle that's being looked at. A person suffering from ON is characterized as a person who has a very restricted diet due to unrealistic fear.

While most people who suffer from ON are trying to eat a healthy diet, their diet becomes anything but healthy as their disorder progresses and they remove more and more foods from their diet.

Unlike anorexia nervosa, people with ON don't worry about the amount of food or calories they consume. Their concern is about what they are eating. This is a life choice to focus on food which has gotten out of control and become an obsession or compulsion.

It may appear to the average lay person that all 'granola loving hippies' suffer from this disorder. But that's not necessarily true. A person with ON has lost the ability to make choices for themselves. They are paralyzed by fear of the same foods most people, even granola loving hippies, consume without hesitation.

The question an ON person may ask the average person is, "Why aren't *you* also afraid of the foods you're eating?" To them, most food is to be feared and avoided.

A day on Facebook, reading all of the memes about evil, giant agri-businesses and chemical corporations, reveals a lot of information and misinformation about the global food supply.

These spark conversations among both the informed and ill-informed. To a person dangerously close to or entrenched in ON, those conversations can be dangerous. They become even more fearful after a day of reading these posts.

So, although ON is translated as literally "correct appetite," it is actually an out of control obsession with what a person eats. "Correct" becomes impossible to achieve and a person puts more and more restrictions on their diet as their compulsion worsens.

2. How are people diagnosed?

A standard diagnostic questionnaire has been developed to help diagnose healthy eaters who have taken things too far:

1. Do you care more about the virtue of what you eat than the pleasure you receive from eating it?

2. Does your diet socially isolate you?

3. Do you spend more than 3 hours a day thinking about healthy foods?

4. When you eat the way you're supposed to, do you feel in total control?

5. Are you planning tomorrow's menu today?

6. Has the quality of your life decreased as the quality of your diet increased?

7. Have you become stricter with yourself?

8. Does your self-esteem get a boost from eating healthy?

9. Do you look down on others who don't eat this way?

10. Do you skip foods you once enjoyed in order to eat the "right" foods?

11. Does your diet make it difficult for you to eat anywhere but at home, distancing you from family and friends?

12. Do you feel guilt or self-loathing when you stray from their diet?

Answering 'yes' to just two of the above questions would diagnose a person with at least a mild form of orthorexia nervosa.

3. Who suffers from Orthorexia Nervosa?

As described previously, ON people have come under the scrutiny of mental health professionals due to their interest in eating as healthy a diet as possible.

According to news sources, people who suffer from the disorder are those who obsess over the foods they put into their bodies.

They try to find only organic, non GMO foods in grocery stores and at farmers markets. Most spend hours a day shopping for and planning means.

These people will often forgo family gatherings and potlucks as well as restaurant eating. If they do attend, they will bring a container with their own food in it or refuse to eat anything.

The people who have this disorder are not hard to spot. Doctors say they suffer from obvious weight loss. They also talk about their food preferences and may seem arrogant as they discuss their clean lifestyle, healthy eating, and avoidance techniques.

4. Where are "Correct Appetite" people hanging out?

Correct appetite people are everywhere. They may be highly educated or high school dropouts. They live in cities, small towns, or on farms. They are wealthy, poor, and middle class.

People who live a healthy lifestyle shop in chain grocery stores but probably not as much as the average person. They may shop mostly at farmers' markets and health food stores.

People with ON will find it impossible to shop at a regular grocery store because of their suspicions about the foods being sold. They may attempt to shop in the same stores most people do but will become paralyzed with fear if there aren't any trusted organic foods available.

If there aren't places for them to shop, they will have more health issues than if they lived near an organic farm or ranch.

Having a very limited availability of acceptable organic foods will cause health issues.

5. What makes them different?

People who suffer from orthorexia nervosa tend to read labels and reject foods that don't meet their stringent standards for purity. Even foods labeled 'organic' may not pass their radar.

They will ask questions about how foods at the farmers' markets were grown, making sure there were no mad-made chemicals involved in any part of the process from farm to farmers' market.

A person with ON has a lot of food and diet rules. They will find a supplier and only use that trusted source.

Some will grow their own vegetables and fruit and raise their own meat animals. While this lifestyle in itself doesn't accurately label a person as having ON, their obsession with perfection will.

Their need to discuss and explain every aspect of their organic garden and severely controlled and restricted diet will quickly give them away.

With the previous questionnaire you can probably accurately diagnose a few people you know who suffer from ON.

But what makes a person with ON different from a person with severe food allergies and / or intolerances?

Speaking from experience, a person with food allergies and intolerances will look to the world like an anorexic or orthorexic (if they are aware of the disorder).

They also have issues with shopping in grocery stores, read labels, reject foods that don't pass inspection, and mimic a lot of the other behaviors of an ON person.

The difference is, while a food sensitive person avoids certain foods for health reasons, they lament and pine for the foods they crave but can't eat. They are not proud of their limited diet; they are ticked off about it.

6. Why do they eat this way?

People who suffer from orthorexia nervosa have a fear of inorganic foods which may contain dangerous or deadly chemical residue. They reject GMO (genetically modified organisms) foods, even if they were raised 'organically.'

They also find their self worth in the foods they eat, as opposed to an anorexic who finds self worth in how thin they can get.

According to psychologists, people limit their eating to the point of poor health because it is impossible to get all of the vitamins, minerals, calories, and essential nutrients in such a severely restricted diet.

The reason they limit their intake is due to fear of pesticides, herbicides, GMO, and unsafe handling and additives during processing. But it's also about control.

They might say they despise corporate greed, and blame them for the use of more and more dangerous chemicals on our foods.

They suffer from an obsessive compulsive personality disorder that reveals itself in the way they eat.

The average person won't be able to understand the mindset of a person with ON. Telling them to relax and eat a hamburger is akin to telling them to drink poison.

7. When did healthy eating become a disorder?

Practitioners are seeing negative effects of extremely restricted diets in patients with ON. These effects include emaciation, malnutrition, and even anorexia, among others.

As explained above, healthy eating isn't the issue. It may be the trigger for the obsessive behavior though. As the disorder progresses, there is nothing healthy about the eating a person with ON is doing.

While they may be eating a lot of something, they are not eating enough of a variety of foods and are missing vital nutrients.

They will also avoid medications for illnesses, choosing natural, homeopathic remedies instead.

A person may or may not realize they have a problem. Family and friends may write them off as weird, crazy, or any number of other insulting descriptions.

8. What do healthy eaters have to fear?

Nothing! According to Bratman, healthy eating only becomes a problem when a person limits their diet to the point of obsessive avoidance.

This leads to the side effects listed above.
As far as health conscious people fearing anything; as long as a person's diet isn't terribly restricted, experts say they are fine. A variety of foods in large enough portions should not cause any problems.

"It's not that I don't support eating healthy food. It's only that when healthy eating becomes an obsession, it's no longer healthy, "says Dr. Bratman.

9. Is there hope?

For people who are concerned about the possibility of an ON diagnosis, there is hope. Eating disorder clinics have programs specifically written for people with orthorexia nervosa.

There are also plenty of psychologists with experience in obsessive compulsive disorders who can treat someone with ON.
As with any addiction, the problem may be in getting to the point of admitting they have a problem.

Family members who are concerned can seek out the advice of a licensed therapist with OCD experience and a good reputation for treating people with ON disorder.

A Bing or Google search will bring up a host of treatment and recovery centers and hospitals.

National Eating Disorders Association has articles with information about this fairly new disorder.

An excellent resource:

www.nationaleatingdisorders.org

800-931-2237

Who cares?

Family members and sufferers care. Eating disorders are difficult to treat and, for the one consumed by ON, difficult to heal from without comprehensive, professional treatment.

People who simply eat a healthy diet have nothing to worry about. As long as you can answer those questions in the questionnaire with mostly "No" you are not in the danger zone.

Thoughts.

As a celiac without an official diagnosis and a person with several severe food allergies, I often carry my own food into restaurants. I also avoid parties and potlucks, sip a cup of tea while everyone else eats at a fast food franchise, and am terrified of food other people prepare for me.

If I had a child with celiac disease with no official diagnosis and several severe food allergies, I would treat her the same way.

Questions about this becoming an official disorder:

- *Would a doctor or psychologist see me restricting the diet of my child for no reason (in his or her mind) and say I'm abusing my child?*

- *Will there be a new diagnosis in the near future for parents with children who suffer from severe food allergies and intolerances;*

   "Orthorexia nervosa by proxy"?

- *Will this diagnosis be used in custody battles between divorcing parents?*

- *Will it be used as an excuse for Child Protective Services to remove children from homes?*

Stay vigilant

&

eat healthy my friends!

www.ingramcontent.com/pod-product-compliance
Lightning Source LLC
Chambersburg PA
CBHW071349310526
45790CB00018B/1403